THE G.I.F.T
GOD INTENDED FOR THIS
By: Jerrell Brown

I hope this book will inspire you, give you the motivation you need to live in your purpose, and pursue what was intended for you.

Acknowledgements

I want to personally thank everyone who has supported me, as well as, those who doubted me. You have all helped me grow into the man that I am today. I want to thank my mom and dad because without them I wouldn't be here. I would also like to thank the beautiful Kara Marie for pushing me to my full potential, encouraging me to pursue my dreams, and showing me what love really is.

Contents

Are you living, or are you simply, existing?
"THE SEED"

I had an idea, not too long ago, to transform my thoughts into words and describe the process I use to accomplish my goals. I am Jerrell Deion Brown, but most know me as Rell, and though I am not an author or even a person who enjoys writing, I thought it'd be best to share with you this gift that has been granted to me because it is not only my gift, but yours as well. I am a fitness and health expert, who eats, breathes, and dreams about the gym. I also think about the many ways it can enhance the lives of all of us. I am 22 years young, so I have a long way to go before I am where I want to be in regard to my expertise in fitness and health management, but I have seen that setting a strong foundation paves the way for unimaginable accomplishments.

My favorite rapper, Lil Wayne, once said,

"some say greatness gets better with time,"

and over my span of life I've seen that "time" is the most important asset we have. However, it is what we do with our "time" that sets the tone for our lives. I imagine the majority of you all are wondering which direction I plan on taking this idea of "time." For starters, if time is our biggest asset, then the tools we use and the amount of effort we put in during each period of time will then determine our outcomes. Life does not give you what you want, it gives you what you deserve.

I challenge you to take a step back for a moment to admire the Chinese bamboo tree. In its physical appearance, the bamboo tree does not look nearly as big or strong as other trees, like sequoias, oaks, and sycamores. Bamboo trees are slim and they do not even bear any flowers or fruit. However, bamboo trees are primarily the only trees still rooted in the ground after raging storms, harsh winters, and extreme summers. Even some of the world's largest and tallest trees cannot withstand certain conditions that the bamboo tree can. The bamboo trees resilience can be traced back to its foundation. To grow a Chinese bamboo tree, a seed is planted in the ground and each day, for five years, the seed is watered and fertilized, but does not ever break the surface of the ground. After five years pass, the bamboo tree grows up to 90 feet tall in only five to six short weeks. So then the question arises, did the bamboo tree take five years or six weeks to grow?

In order for the bamboo tree to break the ground, it needed a strong foundation. In order for it to withstand storms that other trees couldn't, it needed to be deeply rooted. Finally, in order for the tree to be all that the eyes can see, it needed time. It takes five years for a bamboo tree seed to be recognized as more than just a seed. Bamboo tree seeds are like the seeds we plant in our own lives. Regardless of your goals in life, the seeds that you plant in order to help you achieve them, require time. You can not expect nature or some other cosmic force to grow a seed for you. In order to plant an effective seed, you need purpose. You will use this purpose to build a foundation that will ground you and keep you deeply rooted in all of your goals in life, much like the bamboo tree. Time will allow you to build foundations that will lead you to success in life. Time will also allow you to develop your purpose, which will lead to your goals being attained.

When you plant your idea seed, you have to feed it with time, passion, commitment, consistency, and dedication for it to grow and be seen. Things like this don't happen overnight, so you have to be patient and set short term and long term goals.

Short Term Goals:

____
____
____
____
____
____

Long Term Goals:

____
____
____
____
____
____

Fitness is more than just trips to the gym for me, it is my whole life. Some people might not understand why I have such a strong connection to fitness because they are not in my shoes, much like how I might not fully understand their passions or careers. However, that is what this book is about. I intend for this book to give you all an inside look into my life and show you all how fitness relates to everyone's life in so many ways. This book is also intended to be a motivating tool that helps you chase your dreams and never give up, even if you fall short.

My clients often ask,

"when will I see results?"

as if I'm a fitness god and that with the snap of my fingers they will accomplish all of their fitness goals. This is not the case and, most times, I tell them that they will begin to notice results around eight weeks in and that their fitness abilities will get better over time. As a fitness expert, my focus is the gym and the work you put in when I'm with you, but what really counts is what you do with the time when you are outside of the gym. Will you be dedicated and have the discipline to be great or will you give in and continue to be the same person you were and cheat yourself? Consistency is key. In order to reach your fitness and life goals, you have to be consistent with the work you put into your diet and exercise regimen. It's all about the hours that you are not in the gym that determine the results that you get and the rate you get them. It is my job to give you the blueprint to get in shape, but it is your job to continue to workout and eat healthy when I am not around. Many times the ones who cheat themselves are the ones who come running to me crying that they don't have any results.

When this happens, my first question is,

"Did you stick to the diet plan?"

and most times the answer is always the same, "no." People have a hard time discontinuing their bad eating habits, but still expect their physical appearance to change. A famous quote in the fitness world is,

"Don't complain about the results you didn't get for the work you didn't do."

How do you expect to move forward if your mindset and behavior stay the same? It's like pressing the gas when the car is in park. The engine will run, the car will make noises, and if you listen from a distance it may sound like the car is going fast, but in reality, it has not moved. You have to change gears and put the car in drive to be able to go, meaning that to move forward you need to take action. Some of my clients come to me wanting to drop a few pounds in a week or are trying to slim down in preparation for an upcoming holiday or birthday. People fail to understand that fitness is a lifestyle and that it is both, mental and physical. Your mindset has to fit the goals you verbally speak out loud.

"Actions speak louder than words"

You can tell me what you want to accomplish, but will the actions that you show match up with the words you choose to speak? On various times, people have asked me,

"What do I have to do to look like you, Rell? ", "I want to be like you when I grow up, Rell ," or "What's your secret?."

I am 22 years old and I have been working out since I was 15. That equals to seven years of uninterrupted gym time, day-in and day-out grinding, and putting in work so I could be better than the day before. To look how I look today, it was a process. I didn't just snap my fingers and wake up like this. That is not how life works. I didn't get like this in one day, and neither can you. As I previously said, life does not give you what you want, it gives you what you work for. The same people asking me "what is your secret?" Didn't see the seven years of me consistently lifting and going to the gym. People just see the now and not the seed that I planted. They weren't there to see me feed it with consistency and determination. Everyone now sees the product of my hard work. So with that, I tell you that this thing takes time. The Chinese bamboo tree takes five years to be noticed by nature. So whatever dream you have, don't give up on it. Keep giving it everything you have because you never know when your time will come.

Purpose

What is purpose?

noun,
1. the reason for which something is done or created or for which something exists.
synonyms: motive, motivation, reason, grounds
verb,
1. have as one's intention or objective.
synonyms: intend, mean, aim, design

I didn't always know my purpose in life and I am still figuring it out more and more each day. Hopefully, I discover more of what my purpose is while writing this book. I never imagined that I would tell my story by writing a book. I do know that everyone on this earth has a gift. The first thing I try to instill in the people I train is that they all have purpose. My tagline has always been and will always be: The G.I.F.T.

The G.I.F.T means (G)od (i)ntended (f)or (t)his, "this" being for us all to have a purpose. Do you know that God has purposeful intentions just for you? If you didn't, I'm here to tell you that he does and that you are amazing and have greatness within you. In life, everyone has a special gift that was given to them to fulfill and, no matter what it maybe, it is our duty to obtain each reward that is manifested by walking in our purpose. You must keep in mind that your gift was made especially for you and you alone. If you take hold of your purpose in life, you will have the opportunity to share that piece of you with the world -

which is your 'gift'. It is your job to discover your gift because this is the only way that you will be able to live in your purpose, as well as, share your gift with the world. They say the richest place in the world is the graveyard. Why? It could be because people just exist and they don't live in their purpose. Many people may take their gift to the grave because perhaps they are fearful or will never learn how to express their gift. People will rather go with the flow and accept what is given to them, rather than rebel against the status quo. You have to pass up good to be great and I want to be amazing.

My gift is fitness. It is something that I have always been good at. Fitness feels natural to me and I enjoy each moment of pushing my body to new levels I never saw possible. When I began training, I realized that it was more than just fitness that was my calling, and I'm sure other trainers can say the same. It was about being able to change someone's life, giving them hope, and changing their view and lifestyle. I encourage people to not just be better physically, but mentally, as well. I also encourage them to be an all-around better individual. My job as a Personal Trainer is the greatest job in the world, if you ask me, and I wouldn't trade it for anything. I meet people from different backgrounds, with different skills, and with so many different personalities and mindsets. By spending days and days and countless time with these individuals in the gym, I have the opportunity to learn a lot about them. I get to know them by conversing during our sessions and every story they tell me is unique in its own way. Some people pour out their heart to me the first day at the gym and, usually, they vent about why they want to get in shape or be active. People may want to get active because they see the ways it can change their lives or it can be, as simple as, they just want to look good in the different clothes they have. Some people's stories have nothing to do with the gym and, to them, it's just a comfortable place for them to vent. Everyone's story is different and I have the privilege to hear each and every story, as well as, the opportunity to impact their life and give them hope. Many of my clients have had insecurities about their appearance and they were pretty good at hiding it in their everyday life. They confide in me and tell me their insecurities because they trust me. They feel that they can tell me things that they can't tell anyone else. For most clients, I am a complete stranger and I have the honor of being able to help them feel comfortable with their own body. I don't train people just for money. Even though training is how I make my living, I do not charge crazy high numbers like some trainers who look like they have never even worked out a day in their life. I also don't do it just to help people lose weight. Losing weight is an important part and I do want my clients to reach the goals they have for themselves, but my main and most important purpose is to change their lives, give them new hope, give them confidence, and give them a new lifestyle. I am able to feed their mind with positivity and to provide them with a space that is comfortable for them. Life will put you through some things that will test you and knock you down, but your purpose is the reason that you get back up. It's also the reason you don't give up and continue to fight for your dreams and aspirations.

Why do you do what you do?

____

____

____

Who do you do it for?

____

____

____

____

Answer the above questions and never forget why you started. Always find the positive when life puts you in a negative situation. You have full control over your life

Favorite life Quote:

____

Getting started

Now I am going to tell you the story of how I became Rell the Trainer. I am going to keep it short and sweet because as I stated earlier, I am not an author, nor do I know where this book will go. I am not here to tell you an autobiography about my life, but I am here to help you change your life and show you how fast your life can change and go in a direction you never thought it could go. Much like the Chinese bamboo tree, we must all realize that we all have a purpose in life.

My dad introduced me to fitness at a young age. I started my fitness journey by doing push-ups and playing football. During my high school years, I was always in the gym, mainly working out with my football teammates and some of the security guards at my high school. I had a trainer in ninth grade for about a month or so before I got in trouble with my dad, which resulted in him not paying for my training any longer. I never thought about becoming a personal trainer and I always wanted to be in the FBI or to work for the Secret Service. When I graduated high school and enrolled in college, I majored in criminal justice. My first semester of college, I was on crutches because I tore my ACL from a high school football injury. In my early college days, many of the people I met were through the crutches I used to help me walk around campus. After I healed and no longer needed the crutches, I wore a brace and started exercising more and working out at the gym on my college campus. As I worked out more, I began to gain my muscles and strength back. In 2013, I wasn't as big as I am now, but for a 17-year-old college student, I was considered swole. Most people assumed that my major was sports science because I was always spending my time in the gym. Ladies would ask if I could help them in the gym because they saw the work that I would put in and figured that I knew what I was doing. Out of the few people I had working out with me, only a couple stayed before falling off and not taking the gym life seriously. In my sophomore year in college, I had only trained a few ladies, many of whom only came to the gym occasionally.

I had a good friend named Kiana who called me one day when we were home for winter break and suggested that I start my own personal training business so I could help the people on campus who wanted to work out, but didn't know how or where to start. From that conversation with my friend, I came up with the name "Rellesttraining". The named derived from using my first name, Jerrell, and using it as a play on words with "real", since I pride myself in always keeping it real. The name of my business sounded corny to some people, and it still might, but it caught on. From there, I made a Twitter account for my business and began searching for clients. As time went on, I began to build a decent size clientele and started getting my name out there with the help of many of my clients that showed results over time. It was one client, Samaya, who was pretty skinny when she first came to me but gradually became thicker, which lead to her results going viral on social media. From there, "Rellesttraining" took off and I went from having an average of 20 clients a semester to over 100 clients a semester. Telling you all some of my story will help you all get a better understanding of myself, and of how my business came to be. There's a quote that I like that says,

"you don't have to be great to get started, but you do have to get started to be great".

If we just take a leap of faith, this will solidify the first step in what it takes to living in your purpose. Sometimes, all you have to do to grow your wings is to just get started. So here's to just getting started! To fail is to succeed.

"For I know the plans I have for you, declares the Lord. Plans to prosper you and not to harm you, plans to give you hope and a future." and

"No weapon formed against me shall prosper"

are both quotes from the Bible and explain that at times you will go through hard times or a struggle, but the hard times will pass. God didn't say the weapons wouldn't form, what He said was that they will not prosper. Failure and struggle are the prerequisites to greatness. Embrace the struggle because, soon, you will see there is beauty in it.

So, why are so many people still afraid to fail? The reason is because they have become so mentally weak that when they fail once, they automatically give in and give up. People don't understand that in order to win and succeed, failure is a necessary requirement. Failure might repeat itself multiple times, but eventually you will succeed. If it was intended for you to be great, there are certain obstacles and requirements that you have to endure in order to reach the top of the mountain.

On your journey to greatness, you have to remember that your G.I.F.T is special to you and that it's handcrafted with your name on it. You must strive to be in your own lane and on your own road. A lot of people are in competition with others, want what others have, and become jealous because they don't have it and don't realize that what that person has is not meant for them. Each person's purpose and gift is for them and you have to ask yourself why would you want what someone else has when you can have your own. This is what causes most people to lose sight of their dreams and then, fail. They fall and never get back up because they are chasing something that they can never reach and they are trying to live out someone else's dream. People always ask for more despite not being able to handle what is already on their plate now. The Bible says,

"If you are faithful over a few things, then I will make you ruler over many".

The goal is to focus on what you have now, and later you will be able to master many levels. Fail in order to succeed. Fail until you become great at something, and then move to the next level. Success does not happen overnight and you will be a fool if you believe that it does. There is a quote that says "Everything that you want is on the other side of fear". Do you have what it takes to push through and get to the other side of your fear? Are you willing to put in the effort, to never stop grinding, to exceed all expectations and limitations, and to prove everyone who has ever doubted you wrong?

When I first started training, I remember having a boot camp. The plan was to charge $5 a person, but then I thought, "Who am I? I am just starting out so I'm going to make it free to just get my name out there and get people to come". I posted the boot camp flyer on all of my social media accounts, I told my parents to post it, and I told my parents to tell their friends.

The day of the boot camp, five people showed up. One was my friend who was going to help run the boot camp with me, two were my mom and my dad, and the last two were my two friends who rode there in the car with me. Nobody showed up to this boot camp and I could have gave up then, but I kept doing it. As time went on, the size of the boot camp grew to 12 people, then to 20, and then to 30 people. The biggest turnout I've had for my boot camp so far has been in the 50s and the most people that have registered to come was around 80. I could have gave up and said nobody is supporting me and nobody cares about working out. I could have went back to my dream of having a 9 to 5 job with the FBI or Secret Service. However, I kept pushing and didn't give in.

Right before winter break, I remember telling Samaya, a client and friend, that I needed more clients because I only had about 20 people paying only $30 a month and the money wasn't steady because sometimes clients didn't come back the next month. The following semester, she posted her before and after pictures of her results and it went viral only four months later. What If I gave up after that conversation that we had before winter break and came back into the new year and new semester looking for a part-time job instead of continuing to train and build my business? What if I gave up not knowing that all I had to do was wait four more months and my business would triple in size? What if I would have thrown it all away? Sometimes you are closer to success than you think you are and you just have to stick in there and put up a fight until you reach the level of success that you are striving for. Success is not something that happens to you. It happens because of you and the amount of work that you are willing to put in.

There is a poem called "Struggle" and it says,

"When things go wrong as they sometimes will
When the road you're trudging seems all uphill
When funds are low and debts are high
When you want to smile but you have to sigh
When care is pressing you down a bit
Rest if you must but don't you quit
Success is failure turned inside out
The silver tint to the clouds of doubt
You never can tell how close you are
It may be near when it seems so far
So stick to the fight when hardest hit
Its when things go wrong
That you mustn't quit"

"Tragedy and trials come to everybody, but only the strong survive"

Keep pushing
There is growth in failure. Our job is to learn from it, grow from it, and to take advantage of it. Because next time, you will only be better than you were in the beginning. If you fail and give up, you will regret it later. You might feel the need to settle, but then you realize you don't like your job or the way your life is turning out. If you make a change, you might struggle in the beginning, but at least you are working towards

something that you love and not stuck forever in a place you don't want to be. Follow your dreams and watch them come true. No struggle, no progress. Make the hard choices now, so later your life can be easy. Most people make the easy choices now, and as a result, their lives are harder later. Never forget that there is greatness inside of you.

The Grind

The part of life that people don't appreciate, the part that is most important, the part people are afraid of, is the grind. It's the process that puts you on top. The grind is what makes success feel so satisfying. The grind is knowing that you grinded day in and day out to reach that next level you were aiming for and when you reached it there is no better feeling. Most people just see success and want it, but they don't want to go through the process or put in the time to get there. For me, as a trainer and entrepreneur, the grind is 24/7 and many people can't or just don't understand that lifestyle. I put a lot of time and work into my craft. Is it easy? No, but I'm sure you heard the saying,

"If it was easy, everyone would do it"

The Grind is where you find the glory and where you show the world that you won't back down or take no for an answer. Some people hear the word "no" and they fold and give into the limitations of others. Don't be the person who always runs from a challenge or is just comfortable with being average. Step up to the plate and accept the challenge because if you run now, you will run later and it will become natural or a habit of life. Running away from struggle will leave you with regrets and it will leave your "gift" and dreams in the graveyard. You will have a much better life if you go towards the fight and never back down. Your journey isn't over until you say it's over.

I have always been the type to figure things out on my own and I never really just accepted handouts. I like to work for mine because it feels better when I earn something. The victory is much sweeter that way. I'm not saying I don't ask for help sometimes because everyone needs a helping hand at some point, but the victory is sweeter when you put in the effort. It's appreciated more when you work hard for it and you see all the work pay off in the end. Knowing what it is like to work for what you have is great because it's impossible to lose that feeling. Even if you were to go broke, if you have the "grind" and the mindset, you have still succeeded because having those two things is the true measure of success. A lot of people lose sight of that and they think money is the most important thing in the world. They think money brings happiness, but I'm here to tell you that all the best things in life are free. The most important things in life are things that you can't find in the store or on the shelf because they do not have a price tag on it.

A person who did not grind to become rich and wealthy would be lost and confused if they lost all of their wealth because they would not know what to do or what steps to take because they did not have to work for it in the first place. At this moment, I'm nowhere near where I want to be in life and I don't have all the money in the world, but I am successful. During your life journey, the goal of being successful might change. One day your idea of success might be to open up your own business and the next day it could be to donate to the community. Every time you set out to achieve a goal and complete that goal, it is success.

I had to grind to get where I am today and I had to grind to get my client number to increase from 20 clients to over 400 clients. I am only three years into the game and the impact that I've made is greater than any dream I could have ever thought of. This process has taught me to dream big and every morning when I wake up I pray and ask for God to watch over me and help me become the best trainer in the world. What most people don't understand is achieving success is all mental and that seeing is believing.

"When you see the invisible, you can do the impossible"

I had to prove to my current and potential clients that I was qualified and could lead them during their fitness journey. I had to grind to become a sponsored athlete. I had to grind in order to make business moves and secure business deals. I did all of this with no real experience. Trust me when I say that the grind will never go unnoticed if you are truly grinding like you say you are. Some people fake the grind and talk the talk, but they don't walk the walk. Which one are you? Do you fake the grind on social media? Do you fake it for your friends? Do you do it so you can look cool or are you really putting in the work, day in and day out? Each day, I leave my house around 5:30 AM and do not return home until 8:00 PM. Throughout the entire day, I am on the move and do not take any breaks in between. If you are living in your purpose, then the "grind" should excite you. Getting out of bed in the morning should excite you, but many people love sleep more than they love the grind. They love sleep more than they want to be wealthy. They love sleep more than they want to make a difference. Getting the day started should excite you. Your week should be just as exciting, if not better, than your weekend. You should be hungry and ready to take on the day. You must always remember what you are grinding for and why you are grinding.

I am planning on releasing an app and it should be released by the time you read this book. I encourage you to go download my app, titled The GIFT because it will be the best fitness app on the market. At this specific moment it is April 3rd, 2018, and as I am writing this book that you are now reading, I have boot camps occuring on different college campuses in North Carolina. Soon I'll have boot camps in Texas and Los Angeles. I am able to do this because I have met many people in the fitness industry who were willing to collaborate with me. I have partnerships with a variety of companies and I sponsor many products. Nobody ever taught me how to do any of this, but I achieved it because of the "grind". I have failed many times while on my journey and I may fail more in the future, but that will not stop me from achieving what i want in life and getting what is intended for me. It's in my plan and it is constructed for me. Nobody can stop what God has planned for you.

"I can do all things through Christ who strengthens me"

Effort is between you and you. Nobody can stop you if you are willing to put in the work, willing to grind, and willing to be the best version of yourself.

Colby is a good friend of mine and talking to him is like talking to an old man. He always has wise words and is very deep. We started college the same year and watched each other grow. His work ethic and consistency in his craft is unmatched. I always ask Colby to to connect me to different people or organizations because he has planted a lot of seeds along his journey and has connected with so many people. He is living out his purpose and has been grinding day in and day out. This results in him having the most connection and resources than anyone I know. He has impacted so many people through his efforts and demeanor. It's amazing to see him living in his dream and seeing what God has intended for him.

"Outwork Everyone"

is my motto and it is not because I think I'm better or greater than anyone or feel like I'm on top of the world. It's my motto because "out work everyone" is a simple reminder that no matter how much bigger a person is compared to me, when comparing endurance during weight training, strength, or stamina while working out, no one can out work me. I have a lot of hearth and I have put in so much effort to get to where I am today, so I refuse to be out worked by anyone. My grind and heart are so strong that I truly believe that I can do anything I put my mind to.

On my right arm I have a tattoo that says, 'eat greedy'. This doesn't mean to eat all the food that is in your kitchen. It means that when it comes to life, you must make the best out of any situation that is on your plate and you must work extremely hard to accomplish your goals. You have to keep eating until all of your goals are accomplished, and even when that has happened, the grind never stops because there will always be another thing out there for you to accomplish or learn. A lot of people don't understand that if you have a goal that you envision for yourself, you believe that you can achieve that goal, and you work towards achieving that goal, then you will succeed. That dream has no other choice, but to come true.

The grind is 24 hours a day, 7 days a week, and 365 days a year. When you master the grind, you will be unstoppable. You must truly believe that you can do all things and you can't stop eating until you accomplished everything you have set out to do, and even then, you need to go back for seconds. When you truly believe that you are great and amazing, then you will become unstoppable. So, you have two choices. You can either live your own dreams out or you can be used as a pawn to help someone accomplish their dream. The choice is yours. The goal is not the issue or problem because all things are possible to accomplish. The issue is your actions that get you to accomplishing that goal. Any goal can become a reality if you grind to outwork everyone.

Be yourself

One thing I pride myself in is being who I am and not pretending to be something I am not and I believe others should feel and be the same way. I think everyone should show the world their unapologetic selves and not hold back. I think everyone should own their greatness and believe that they were built to be great. At times, I think people should adjust their personality based on the environment or situation that they're in, but it should still be real, authentic, and 100% who they are. For example, the manner in which you talk to your friends may not be the same way you would talk to your significant other, but both of those sides of you would still be you.

I believe that if someone cannot accept me for who I am, then me and that person could not work well as friends, associates, or business partners. Most people who can't accept you for you, may have their own insecurities or may be jealous of what you have or your potential of what you could be. I'm Rell and will always be Rell. I do not act or try to be anyone else and I think everyone should carry themselves that way, as well. I think everyone should remember that God made them how they are and they do not have to change or conform to anyone else.

I personally don't like to dress up in suits, slacks, button-downs or any other clothes that are considered formal or business attire. In these clothes, I feel uncomfortable. I always prefer to wear a t-shirt and sweatpants, unless it's absolutely necessary for me to dress up. The perception of those who wear business attire or formal wear is that the person is sophisticated, intelligent, and professional. Some jobs require you to wear business or business casual at the workplace and I understand why, but it's definitely not my taste. When I do dress up, I must admit that I do look sharp, but the clothes I wear or the material things I have do no interest me. I'm interested in the connections that I make and the knowledge that I obtain, especially when I'm conducting business, networking, or just casually talking to someone. I don't think I need a suit and tie to show someone that I'm professional. I believe that I can wear a tank top and shorts and still display that I am knowledgeable. Unfortunately, in certain situations, if you don't look the part or fit someone's standards you'll get overlooked.

It's important to not judge a book by its cover by focusing on clothes or material items. People should value the conversations that are being had and learning from one another. I don't care if someone looks "professional" because, to me, professionalism does not have a look. Professionalism is a mindset and it's all about actions and conduct.

For example, as a trainer, a lot of my clients are women and some of them are attractive. In the past, I would flirt with some, build small relationships, but not really build anything serious with them. This would hurt my business because some of the women would become upset if I didn't want anything serious with them and some women would get jealous when they found out that I was pursuing other women. In both of these situations, the women would not want anything to do with me and cancel their training sessions. On the other side, some women who were my clients that I pursued would believe that just because we were hanging out meant that they would receive free training sessions. These situations made me quickly realize that I needed to be more professional and not handle my business like that.

This brings me to a story that further explains my point. When I was in my senior year of college, I met another physical trainer who was probably in his 30s. He wanted to collaborate with me so we met up during my homecoming week at school. He found out about Rellest Training through word-of-mouth marketing and he told me that people told him a lot about me. We met up again that next week to talk business and things were going well because we both had good ideas. With him being older, he had been in the fitness industry longer than I have so I was learning a few things from him. The conversation then starts becoming weird and going downhill because he begins to mention sexual acts and relationships he experienced with his women clients. At first, I wasn't too concerned because I thought we were just talking as guys, but then as it continued, I became concerned. I started to re-think doing business with this man because he was unprofessional, and that was just unacceptable, especially for someone who was around 10 years older than me.

 A few months later, I decided to look past how unprofessional he was and give him a chance. We had a business idea of hosting a New Year's boot camp that would be open to the whole city. At the time, I was working with a trainer who was a woman. She was really cool and had a bright future ahead of her. One day, we all meet up for a meeting and during the meeting the 30-year-old trainer was flirting with the woman trainer and making her feel comfortable. When the woman trainer went out to take a phone call, the 30-year-old trainer asked me if her and I had any history. I immediately became frustrated with him because we were at a business meeting and not on some type of weird blind date. Professionalism is about carrying yourself in a manner that makes people want to work with you. It's not about how you look, it's about portraying professionalism from the inside. After that meeting, I never talked to or did business with that guy again because he put my business partner in an uncomfortable setting. He couldn't move past his sexual thoughts to be able to conduct real business that might impact many people in a positive way.

As a college student, I learned that networking was really important. I, personally, don't care much for schoolwork and, in my case, I feel that school is like a scam to get our money. School is a cycle of teachers feeding students information, students studying the information for a test, and then the students taking the test and forgetting what they've learned. There's rarely any real teaching and learning happening in the classroom. The cycle is not setup for most students to retain the information for a long period of time. Schools cares more about grades than they do about whether or not the student actually learned or retained the material and knowledge. A lot of students cheat in college because information is being taught very quickly and it does not give students enough time to retain and learn it properly. Also, at times, the professors don't allow for students to actually apply the information that is being taught. Usually, the professor just stands at the podium, reads off the PowerPoint slides, and then the students just listen and, then go home. The education system and the manner of how teachers conduct classrooms can use some improvement. It doesn't make sense to pay thousands of dollars to be taught in this manner when I can just google this same information for free.

Society has held college to a very high standard. It is presented as a place that is a requirement to attend in order to get a job, however, a lot of people who have jobs now are working in fields that are not relevant to their college major. A lot of people either grow to not like their major and were in too deep to change it or a lot of workplaces just don't care about the career field you studied in college. The quote, "It's not what you know, but who you know" is very relevant in many situations like this. For example, there might be two people applying for a job and one has a 3.8 GPA, and the other has a 3.2 GPA. The job they're applying to may choose the person with the 3.2 GPA because the person has a connection with someone who already works for that establishment. Is it fair? To some, it is and to others, it isn't. Personally, I think it is fair because if the hiring manager knows an applicant, then they know their character and work ethic. I don't think that a GPA is an appropriate measure of knowledge. For me, it's not a credible source. Some people may or not agree with me on this subject, but it's fine because I am trying to introduce a different perspective.

In college and high school, teachers should teach students about topics like managing money, buying a house, paying student loan debt, and etc. These are basic things that most people need to know to be successful. Everyone eventually wants to know how to buy a car, buy a house, or save and invest money, but most people don't know how. We invest a lot of money into our educations, but do not learn basic life skills. For example, in college, I was enrolled in a environmental science class where I learned about climate, soil, and rocks. As a personal trainer, this was a subject I didn't need to learn about. I couldn't care less about a rock or a certain kind of tree. I would've preferred to spend my time and money on learning about things that would be beneficial to me later, such as filing taxes while owning your own business. The educational system might not teach students things like this because maybe it wants students to just be an employee their whole lives or live a safe life and not dream or live life to the fullest. Most people do not have financial intelligence, which may be the reason why a lot of people are in debt today.

If people who have graduated from college were asked to return to college and retake old tests, they would probably fail. College is designed for students to remember material to pass a test and after college, most people don't even remember half of the things that college taught them. However, what most people do remember is the people they met along the way, the connections they made, the friendships they formed, and that the experiences they shared with these people would last a lifetime. This is the most important part of college. Utilizing these connections are also important. I think students should spend their time in college being involved in clubs and organizations, networking, and meeting new people because they can learn so many things from these people who have various backgrounds and experiences. You never know who you might need later down the road or who might need you. As a trainer, my clients have a variety of skills and professions. The professions that my clients have include, making clothes, doing eyelashes, doing hair, creating meal prep plans, and etc. I am blessed to have such a diverse network. I also help others by connecting them to people I know.

Self love is very important. The more you love yourself, the more comfortable you are with being uncomfortable. When God puts you in a uncomfortable situation, that means it's your time to grow. Some people might think self love is cocky, but I see it as having confidence. I don't think anyone should feel higher than anyone else because we are all created equal, but I do think people should be confident in who they are as a person, know their worth, and know the things that they have to offer to the world. People should have swag in their talk and walk. They should be able to be confident in how they show the world who they are and they should not hold back. Everyone might not like you, but that's okay because life is about being comfortable within your own skin, despite the environment or who is watching.

Never look back

In life, everyone has things they might or might not be ashamed of. Everyone has a past. Most people have secrets only they know and that they will take with them to the grave. The past is the past for a reason and you can't dwell in it. If you live in the past you will never grow. You have to live in the moment and look towards the future. Focusing on the present is most important. Life is all about what you make out of the 24 hours that you have each day.

How do you spend your time?
What are you doing to do succeed?

Even though you are supposed to focus on the present, don't be afraid of your past. You should embrace it because it is the reason you are who you are today and every experience in your life, good or bad, impacted you somehow. Every moment in your life had a purpose, which got you to where you are today. God inserts people or situations into your life for a greater good in the future.

When I was in high school, I tore my ACL. I also wanted to play football on a college level, but God had other plans for me. One day at practice in my senior year of high school, I tore my ACL and I just knew I would never be able to play football again. The next year, it was time for me to choose which college I wanted to go to, but I didn't know what college to choose. When planning for college, I always told myself that football would help me get into college and choose which college to go. However, with football out of the picture, I was lost and confused.

College was never a big thing in my family. When deciding on which college to go to, my mom told me to go on online to search for colleges that stood out to me, but I really didn't even know what I was looking for. One Sunday when I was going to church with my friend and his family, my friend's mom came to pick me up and was asking me about college. I told her I didn't know where I wanted to go and didn't really have any colleges that interested me. She proceeded to tell me that she attended North Carolina A&T and she loved it. Her stories and experiences at North Carolina A&T was the most information I had ever heard about college. She sounded like she had a great time there so, that day after church I applied to the school. I filled out the application, my mom helped me write my essay, and on Christmas, I got accepted. That moment, I remembered thinking that it was all a sign from God. I learned about North Carolina A&T while on my way to church and I received my acceptance letter on Christmas day.

At the time, I didn't know the reason why God wanted me to go to North Carolina A&T or why he was taking me down that path. I sat in my room and prayed to God asking him if this was the school for me. 5 years later, I am now a graduate from North Carolina A&T. If I hadn't torn my ACL or gone to church that morning with my friend, I wouldn't have been at North Carolina

A&T. God maneuvered me for a greater purpose that I could not see at the time. In my sophomore year at North Carolina A&T, before I started Rellesttraining, I needed a job because I was broke from buying books and didn't want to keep asking my mom for money. I went to the gym and asked one of the employees if I could work there and they said yes and told me to fill out an application. A week later, they gym called and told me that they couldn't hire because they only hired sports science fitness management students and on my application it said that my major was criminal justice.

Maneuvered

I was mad at the time but that's because I couldn't see the bigger plans that God had for me. The next semester, a girl gave me the idea to start training people on my own, which led me to start Rellesttraining. I made a job for myself, since the gym didn't give me one. God still had a plan bigger for me that I couldn't see. A year later in my junior year, I finally decided to switch majors to sports science. My mom was mad because switching majors hindered me from graduating on time and she would have to spend more money. I understood her frustrated, but I was listening to God and I didn't tell my mom about switching majors until after I did it. I wanted to avoid her trying to talk me out of it.

Maneuvered.

By changing my major, I was able to meet and network with people who were in my field. While I was growing and becoming the number one trainer on campus, I began to see how God had this plan laid out for me. I was able to sit on panels and talk about fitness, compete in an entrepreneurial contest, be a mentor to other trainers in my field, and inspire others. This journey all started that day when I tore my ACL and if it wasn't for that moment, I would have never came to North Carolina A&T. If it wasn't for that moment, I would have never applied to the gym and been rejected to work there. If it wasn't for that moment, I wouldn't be where I am today as a business owner and a personal trainer.

Sometimes we have a moment in our life that we think is a defeat, but it is really a victory. When I tore my ACL, I sat in my bed and cried. I felt helpless and I had no idea on what to do next since football was all I knew. I didn't know me tearing my ACL was a blessing and the beginning of my journey to success. I wanted to play football and God redirected my path towards me sharing my gift.

Maneuvered.

So when things don't go as planned in life, don't be so quick to get mad or upset because things didn't go your way. God has something better for you than you have for yourself. God has a greater purpose for you than you have for yourself. If God would have never redirected me, I wouldn't have been able to impact so many lives. I wouldn't have been able to connect and network with so many people. I probably wouldn't even be writing this book and you wouldn't be here reading it. You would be doing something different with your time so maybe this is God's way of showing you something, as well. Everything has a purpose and reason behind it and this book was meant to have some kind of impact on you or God wouldn't have put it into your hands.

Don't limit yourself or your growth as a person. You have unlimited potential and there's always another level that you can reach. Nothing lasts forever and you can always get better. Think of it like a car, such as the more you drive, the more gas you need. You can't live forever off one tank of gas. You have to continuously add more the further you go. This applies to life because the more you chase your dreams, the more you grown. More will be required. Massive thoughts must be followed by massive actions. Set goals so high that even if you don't reach them, you reach something that you may have not even thought was possible. For example, if your goal is to make an extra $1,000 a month, set your goal to make an extra $5,000 a month. If you miss the $5,000 mark and make an extra $3,000 a month, then it's better than your first goal of $1,000.

"Every time I thought I was being rejected from something good I was

actually being redirected to something better"

Network is your net worth

While in college, you will meet people with different backgrounds and work ethics. This even expands outside of college and into life. The saying goes, "birds of a feather flock together" which means people with similar mindsets spend the most time together. If you hang around four broke people, you will soon become the fifth.

Everyone has friends who they hangout with in different situations. People have friends that they party with, friends that they study with, and just everyday friends that they can call whenever to chill. When I first got to college, my whole freshman year involved getting girls and partying all the time. Every Thursday through Saturday, my friends and I went to parties and were focused on living life and enjoying the moment. However, as my college career went on, I gained knowledge, matured, and grew. My mindset began to change. I started to think differently and when I started my business, I faded away from the party scene. I'm not saying I stopped partying all together, but I did cutback a lot. I started to look at parties as places that didn't always offer positive things. For example, at some parties there would be fights, shootings, and people getting too drunk. Some people I know do still party every weekend faithfully and that's cool, but the goal should always be to change and to grow. It is important that people focus on doing positive things with their time so they can have a better tomorrow. There is a saying that says,

"live today like others won't, so you can live tomorrow like others can't."

I agree with this statement 100% because I have seen many of my friends focus only on partying and doing the bare minimum in college just to graduate. They did not make any real connections or have anything to look forward to after college because they did not use their time wisely.

At some point in everyone's life, a person has to determine who they will surround themselves with and ask themselves if certain people contribute to their life in a positive way. People have to decide if some people in their life are an asset or a burden who is deadweight and that they are dragging along. This decision to cut off friends who are burdens may be difficult. In my college career, I encountered some friends who did not benefit my life at all. Many of these people just wanted to drink and smoke all day and chase after girls. However, my interests in doing things like that ended my sophomore year. My focus was all about grinding and having an impact on people's lives. I began to surround myself with people who thought like me and who had similar goals and business ideas. I surrounded myself with people who I could rely on to help me better myself.

My freshman year of college, I almost got into a fight with a guy because I decided not to pay to get into one of his parties. About a year ago, that guy and I recently came in contact with each other because we were both in the fitness field. He used to be a trainer as well, but then he branched off to explore the mental health route. He started a project called, "Trust your Journey", which is now a nonprofit. Seeing his growth in those five year is amazing. We have sat on panels together and worked on similar projects. He is only 22 years old, but he has the soul of someone who is much older and wiser. I'm sure you have a friend or someone you know who is similar to him. Connecting with Colby has benefited me in so many ways because he has gotten my involved in his network and even connected me with a developer for my app. It's people like Colby that I like to connect myself with and be around. I still have my friends that I like to party with and they know and respect that I have a different mindset. At one point I tried to help them change their ways and mindset too, but it's not for everyone. I knew if I stayed around them all day and didn't branch out to explore new things, then nothing would have got done for me.

God also brought another person into my life who has been a huge blessing. That person is my girlfriend who will, hopefully, be my wife one day. One thing that I have learned is that women make the world go around. Some of the most strongest and influential people in my life have been women and they just know how to do so many things. Women are problem solvers and they are a true blessing. Men who are reading this, make sure you cherish the women who are in your life.

My girlfriend's business is called, "Karamarieservices". She designs, styles, and installs wigs. She hopes to expand her business and invest in other services as well. I'm not going to give away all of her secrets. I have known her for about 8 months now and she is the most influential person that I have ever had in my life. She has a great business mind and a drive to go for what she wants. She is always giving me new ideas and helping me with things that I used to just try to figure out myself. She helps me build brand my brand and I try to do the same for her. We have a partnership within our relationship and I love it and am excited to see where it takes us. People always ask why I like her so much and what makes her different. My first response is always that I love her mind because it's amazing. I see how great she is and I know she has greatness in her. Recently, I took my girlfriend and two of our friends to my financial advisor because I believe that we will all become successful business owners in years to come. I am the type who will always look out for others in anyway I can. It's just something that is in me. There is a quote that says,

"As long as you make sure someone else's life is

okay, God will make sure you life is ok."

I love having a network of people that are trying to better themselves and working on their goals. My goal is to try to help them out as much as I can by using the things that I know and have figured out thus far. I love being around positive and impactful people who share a similar vision of grinding and making an impact. Having people like this in your circle is a major key to life because it's added motivation. The people in your circle will constantly look out for one another and are ready to provide you with a connection if you need one. With all of these resources from your network, you can and will develop a bigger net worth.

So, ask yourself if the people you hang out with are conducive to your success. Are they benefiting you or are they holding you back from reaching your potential? Some people might say if someone is holding you back, then you should cut them off. I would not go to that much of an extreme, but I would say you should distance yourself away from them and find people who are contributing to your greatness. You can still have a set of friends for times you want to just party and let loose, but make sure you are always surrounding yourself with positive people and positive energy. Remember, birds of a feather flock together, so if you hang around four millionaires you will soon become the fifth.

Faith

"You can't speed up or slow down the river, so at some point you have to have faith."

"A village all went outside to pray for rain, but only one showed up with an umbrella and that was the one who had faith."

"Walk by faith, not by sight."

In life, you have to live in the moment and cherish each moment because no day is promised. You should always have dreams, have goals, and be passionate about what you want to accomplish. Always be effective and when you're in each moment you should act like your time is almost over. "If tomorrow wasn't promised, what would you give for today?", said Ray Lewis. You should really ask yourself that question and think about it. What would you give if tomorrow wasn't going to come? Time is the most important asset to life, but often it is taken for granted. It's the greatest gift that we are given, but if God didn't limit it would you truly value it? Would you still have the same attitude and the same work ethic? Would you have the same hopeful manner or the same faith if there was no limit on time? Most people would probably say "no" to these questions because with the limited time they have, they don't truly value it.

So, if tomorrow wasn't promised, what would you give today? When you wake up in the morning you have to be efficient with your time and you have to have faith that the things that you're doing today will bring you better days tomorrow. There are people who believe in you and have invested in you. You owe it to them and the world to be efficient with the time you are given. You are a blessing to this world and the world is a blessing to you. Time is the blessing that God gave you. It's the reason you are here. When you don't feel like doing something and push it to the next day and the next day and the next day, eventually, the idea will fade you will never do it. Effort is between you and you. You might be able to lie to the world, but you can't lie to the person in the mirror. Be honest with yourself or you will not make it anywhere in life. You might lie to yourself so much that you start to convince yourself that the lie is actually true. Your bad day today doesn't determine your tomorrow. You have to have faith and you have to be efficient in the way you move and the way you value your time. I made a promise to myself that I would have fitness boot camps on college campuses other than North Carolina A&T. I didn't know how I would do it and I had no idea where to start, but I had faith and God brought the opportunities to me. He blessed me with the chances to be able to get out of my comfort zone and pursue things I hadn't before. I love being able to impact people that I don't even know or might not ever see again. I had faith in my dream and God made it a reality. I had no Idea four other colleges would be calling me and asking me to come to their school to share my gift. However, I did believe that one day my dream would become a reality and that's called faith. It was through my efforts that God made it a reality.

God puts certain people in your life and uses those people to help you grow along your journey. One day, I arrived on campus like any other day and parked in my usual spot. A random guy that I didn't know drove by me in a truck. When he saw me, he stopped and said that he wanted to be like me one day. I get that statement a lot. People always tell me that they want to have a body that looks like mine. I said thanks for his compliment and we laughed and he drove off. I didn't really think too much of it. The next day, I saw the same car when I pulled into the parking lot. It's raining, but I see the guy again and he drove past me. When I was pulling into the parking lot, he honks at me and I honked back. As I got out my car, he stopped and said something out of the window, but I couldn't really hear him so I got a little closer. He told me that God was going to use me and open up doors for me that will allow me to impact others. I was thankful for that and told him, "Oh that's what's up. I really appreciate that." Those words gave me more fuel to my fire. It reminded me to always give 110%. God uses people to give you signs along your journey and since that day, I haven't seen that man in that parking lot since. Those few words that he said to me was something I have not and will never forget.

"You did not create me to worry, you did not create me to fear. You created me to worship daily so I'm

going to leave it all right here."

My friend and gospel artist singer, Anthony Brown, sung those words. I first met Anthony at a concert in Greensboro, NC where he opened up for Kirk Franklin. All of the men in the room were standing up because Kirk Franklin had asked them to. Out of nowhere, I felt a hand on my shoulder and saw that the hand belonged to Anthony Brown. He was the choir director at my church in my hometown, but I had never spoken to him directly. After the concert, we took pictures in the lobby where he was selling his album. Two years later, I am now his trainer and we have been cool ever since. The words that I previously quoted, are words from his song, "Trust in You." When I first heard the song, I thought it was a boring, slow song. I have always preferred faster, upbeat songs. However, as I continued to listen to it, I paid attention to the words and listened to the message of having faith. The song explains that you can't worry about the future and whether or not things happen. You can't be afraid to fail or be scared of life. You can't worry about if you will or will not make it or if you can or cannot handle something. You have to trust in God, trust in your journey, and trust in your gift. You must let go and leave it up to God to handle. You should put in the work and be efficient with your time, but also have faith that everything will eventually workout. Nobody can see the future, so at some point, you have to have faith. If you spend your whole life worrying and being afraid, then nothing will get done.

The next part of the song says,

"I will trust in you, Lord."

You really have to believe in your dreams for them to come true. You have to believe it in your heart and trust in God. That is faith. Imagine if everyone truly believed the verse,

"I can do all things through Christ who strengthens me."

You have to tell yourself every day that you can do all things. When it comes to your dreams, you have to say to yourself, "I can do all things." Imagine if everyone who has ever dreamed truly believed that they could do all things. If so, would the graveyard still be filled with dreams that no one ever heard? Would people still be working the 9-5 job that they hate? Would people who started working on their dreams and gave up because it got hard, still give up? Would we live in a world where they want you to play it safe and work for someone else rather than living your life how you want to live? You can do all things if you believe and have faith. Eventually, it will become a reality. If you believe God's word is true, He will bless you and allow you to walk in your purpose. Check out the song by Anthony Brown "Trust in You". It will change your life.

Make sure you set life goals, yearly goals, monthly goals, and even daily goals. Also, always give 110% for 21 days straight. Don't slack, whether it's in school, your relationship, or in your dreams. Give it all you got for 21 days straight and see if it makes a difference. See if you feel like you found hope in your life and see if you have faith in your dreams that you never had before. The reason you do what you do is most important because it will keep you going. Life will knock you down and if you are weak you will give in. Only the strong survives, so for 21 days remember your why and give 110%. Make a difference and be the change.

My name is Jerrell Brown, CEO Of Rellesttraining, and I hope this book has inspired you and changed your life. Go out and change the world. Live how you want to live. You only have one life so make the best of it.

I think you're an amazing trainer who has done more for me than any trainer that i've trained with. I've seen the most progress while working with you and even though you work with a lot of other people, you make every individuals experience personable. I love that you act like yourself at all times & keep people moving in the gym. You don't force people to come but it's inspiring to see others come without being told. THANK YOU RELL! ❤

-Naomi

Rell is a top-notch, A1 trainer! He has impeccable form and really knows the best exercises, # of reps/sets, and nutrition to help you achieve your goals. Even though the workouts can be grueling--he once had me do 100 deadlifts!--the sessions go by quickly, thanks in part to his sense of humor and candidness. He both challenged and encouraged me to perform exercises I wouldn't have done before. It's damn near magical how I've seen more gainz in the 2 weeks I've trained with Rell than I did in the prior 2 months of training on my own at the gym. So whatever your fitness goals, hit this man up and put in the work. Trust the process.

-Jeff

RELL has not only been my trainer for 3 years but he has and continues to be a great positive male role model in my life. I remember when I first started with him in 2014 I could barely lift a 20lb dumbbell; now I can lift 50 & 60lbs. As a trainer, rell pushes you to your full potential even when you feel like you can't push yourself. He treats all his clients as if we were his own family. Rell is the most blunt & hilarious dude I've ever been around. He has literally turn me into a gym rat which I never thought I would be. There were countless times where I would just come to the gym just to help him out with his other clients and have fun. As of Now I have started my brand as a fitness model thanks to RELL and his crazy training sessions. I went through hell & back to get the results I wanted but it was all worth it! I rarely trust anybody nowadays but RELL is one of the few people that has earned my trust without even trying! Rellesttraining has taught me the meaning of "Believing in yourself" rather than just "success" & "getting big". This is what makes him the best!

~KeithJones
~MrJonesTheModel

If I just appreciate all the hard work you have put into me and helping me reach my goal. it was a great experience and i plan on using what you taught me from here on out. "I gotta eat greedy" is something that will always stick in the back of my hea. So when i feel like giving up, especially when i dont feel like i see results, imma push and eat greedy. appreciate you rell! you are about to change your life by helping others change their lives. In the name of Jesus, I pray He watched over you in your journey and brings many blesses to your door step. love you man!♥keep doing what you do

-Destiny

www.ingramcontent.com/pod-product-compliance
Lightning Source LLC
Chambersburg PA
CBHW031430250726
48656CB00002B/913